The
Schoolwork Success System Handbook

Acknowledgments

Special thanks to Joe Ficek, Paul Kanz, Stacey Mican, Marchelle Watson and Matt Casteel. We couldn't have created this handbook without their constructive feedback and encouragement.

ISBN 979-8690423575

Table of Contents

1. Introduction 5

   Why Use the Schoolwork Success System? 6

   The Schoolwork Success System(S3) Task Board 7

   Supplies...8

   Overview of the Basic Steps 9

2. Block Planning 9

3. Planned Schoolwork: My Assignments 10

4. Final Planning Review 12

5. System Rules 13

6. Today's Schoolwork: My Commitments 14

7. The Morning Stand-up Meeting 14

8. The Target Task 15

9. The Desktop 16

10. Finished Schoolwork: My Achievements..........................17

11. Repeat the Process 17

12. The Schoolwork Success System in Action – An Example 17

10 Tips for Schoolwork Success.......................................31

About the Authors..32

1. Introduction

When Covid-19 appeared in the United States many schools closed facilities then required students to do schoolwork from home. The schools did their best by providing online learning and student portals. However, what schools could not do was provide families clear guidance about how to organize and manage online schoolwork. As the parent of a student, along with thousands of other parents, I did not know where to begin.

After five weeks of doing schoolwork at home, my son, Alan, in the 7th grade at the time, was three weeks away from the end of the schoolyear, and 16 assignments behind! Yikes! Alan and I realized that we needed to figure out a way to reorganize and manage his schoolwork, and do it fast. Alan was getting so many assignments, including having to redo some work, from different teachers and through clicking so many different hyperlinks, that he had a good deal of trouble organizing his assignments, managing his time and tracking his progress. In addition, Alan had been diagnosed with a moderate Attention Deficient Hyperactivity Disorder (ADHD) condition in the 3rd grade, which added to the challenge of staying organized. As a result, Alan and I had to quickly devise a system that would help him succeed.

We created *The Schoolwork Success System* as a practical low-tech, high-touch organizational tool for planning and managing schoolwork at home. It is based on the Kanban methodology developed in the 1940's by Taiichi Ohno for the Toyota Production System. Since then, the concept of visually representing work on a task board to show how work is flowing and tracked, continues to be used successfully in a variety of industries.

Some elements of *The Schoolwork Success System* are based on Agile principles. Agile planning methods break down work into manageable chunks, or tasks and sub-tasks, and then make frequent adjustments to work plans to meet requirements and achieve set goals. Agile emphasizes face-to-face communication through standardizing ceremonial events for making plans, holding meetings and discovering problems. These methods originated in the software development industry but are now widespread in a variety of sectors. Ironically, many companies use low-tech tools for managing high-tech work. Why? Because they can often be more reliable, effective and efficient. *The Schoolwork Success System* is a Kanban-Agile hybrid system that includes a simple, user-friendly task board that is modified to be easily used by parents and students to organize and manage schoolwork. Student's work flow should be smoother, and require less time to manage while parents will be able to simply glance at the board to keep track of the student's progress and quickly identify issues.

Both Alan and I believe *The Schoolwork Success System* will help you and your student organize and manage their online learning experience. The system is designed to help plan and facilitate school workflow, enhance parent-student communication and improve overall academic performance.

Throughout this handbook you will learn about the many features and benefits of *The Schoolwork Success System*. Below is a summary of the key benefits:

Improves Understanding

Students are more likely to understand things that can be touched (tactile) or require movement (kinesthetic) instead of abstract ideas. Organizational and planning activities that include movement often results in reinforcement of memory through the experience of doing something. Students learn more effectively when fine motor movements, such as moving their hands and touching things.

Movement and touch are essential aspects of *The Schoolwork Success System*. Students are required to write down their assignments on sticky notes, and then move the sticky notes around the board in a methodical way. This activity helps improve memory and clarity of what needs to get done and by when.

Improves Organization

Organization does not come easy to most students. It requires a conscious effort, foresight and a great deal of planning; qualities that most students lack. Students often get confused and frustrated with having to keep up and plan for their many classes, assignments, test dates and so forth. Without a good organizational system, students' work and grades often suffer.

The Schoolwork Success System is an effective method of tracking commitments, progress and deadlines. It provides a structured, low-effort, systematic approach to recording necessary information on a daily basis and creates a routine for smoother transitions, less interruptions and a less confusion.

Tracks Achievements

The Schoolwork Success System allows a student to set and track daily and weekly goals. As they accomplish goals and tasks throughout the week, they are able to build momentum and get inspired to work harder. Their confidence increases, work becomes more fluid, and they feel an increasing sense of accomplishment. Goal setting is a great skill to learn for schoolwork as well as succeeding in life.

Enhances Student Responsibility

Having a well-structured system gives students freedom to plan, organize and keep track of their work. This has a dual benefit of increasing the student's accountability to their commitments, and providing them with a structure that will help them achieve success. With *The Schoolwork Success System*, students are able to take full responsibility and be completely accountable for their work.

Creates Awareness

The Schoolwork Success System makes monitoring progress much easier. It is designed to add clarity and awareness for both the student and parent. With the task board, assignments are posted in a highly visible location. There should be no doubt about what needs to get done and by when resulting in increased situational awareness and reduced misunderstandings. By having assignments or tasks on a task board there should clarity on what schoolwork needs to get done and a reduction in missing assignments and other mistakes. Parents can obtain a quick status and remain informed of progress at-a-glance. When problems occur, they are discovered early so action is taken as soon as possible.

Promotes Communication

The Schoolwork Success System serves as an excellent line of communication between students, parents and teachers. It helps clear up any confusion about what needs to get done and by which dates. The system provides scripted talking points so that both parent and student know what to expect each day. By keeping conversations focused and on track, the system encourages participation and buy-in, which can help improve the parent-student relationship and reduce tension. It can show you when the student is struggling, needs encouragement or help with problem-solving, as well where the successes are and when praise is deserved.

The Schoolwork Success System(S3) Task Board

There are two parts to *The Schoolwork Success System:* 1) the S3 Task Board and 2) an easy to follow 10-step procedure. Both must be used together. The S3 Board has nine features that helps schoolwork flow. It uses sticky notes and a workflow structure to visually organize and track the progression of schoolwork, while establishing rules and capturing issues when they occur. The 10-step procedure helps parents and students plan the flow of work, and identify and solve problems, for a given period of time.

The S3 Task Board has the following nine features (see Figure 1):

1. **Priority:** Priorities are the most important things to get done for a given subject, and are most often set by the due dates. The closer the due date, the higher the priority.
2. **Planned Schoolwork:** The work written on sticky notes that is planned to be completed during the designated period of time.
3. **Class Categories:** There are five generic class categories in the Today's Schoolwork area: Social Studies, Math, Science, Language Arts and Music. Additionally, there is a "Class or Meetings" category, for the purpose of creating sticky notes for one-time or reoccurring meetings. Lastly, the "Other" category is for other classes (e.g., electives) that need to be planned and monitored.
4. **Today's Schoolwork:** These are the tasks that the student is committed to complete for the schoolwork needed to be done today.
5. **Block Dates:** Block dates are the start and finish dates of the respective schoolwork planning period, called a block. A block is a time frame in which the next iteration of schoolwork will be planned and accomplished. This is typically a two-week period starting on a Monday and finishing on the Friday after next; although it could be more or less than two weeks, or as long as four weeks. A two-week block of time is recommended.
6. **Finished Schoolwork:** This is where sticky notes of the finished schoolwork tasks are placed when completed.
7. **Rules:** This is a space to write the most important rules that need to be followed to help the student succeed. This could be break times, how priorities are set (e.g., by dates, late work, sequencing, etc.).
8. **Target Task:** This is the "task-at-hand" that should be worked at the moment and be completed first. It is the task the student is working on now.

9. **Desktop:** This space on the board is reserved for tasks or sub-tasks that cannot be completed because something is preventing the student from progressing or finishing the task. This could be a challenging math problem, confusion about the task instructions, or questions for the parent or teacher.

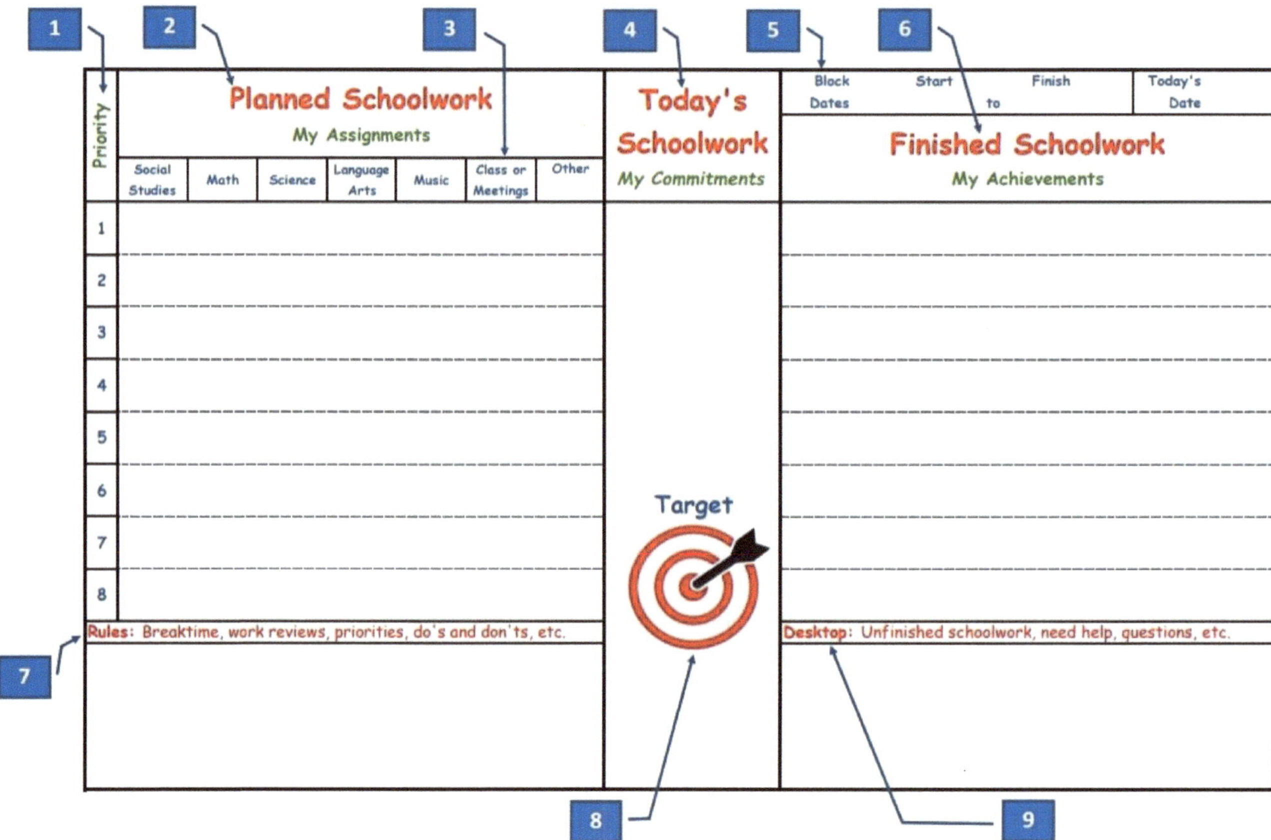

Figure 1

Supplies

These items are needed to effectively use *The Schoolwork Success System*.

<u>Sticky Notes</u>. It is best to have at least four different colors of 1.5" x 2" sticky notes. They can be purchased online or at most department or office supply stores. Using just one color can work too.

<u>Erasable Markers</u>. A fine tipped erasable marker designed for use on a whiteboard can be purchased online or at most department or office supply stores.

<u>Task Board</u>. *The Schoolwork Success System* (S3) Task Board can be made at home or purchased online.

Overview of the Basic Steps

To put *The Schoolwork Success System* into action, follow the 10-step process below in the correct sequence. The remainder of the handbook provides greater detail for each step.

1. Input Block Dates in upper right corner of *The Schoolwork Success System* (S3) Task Board.
2. Collect as many assignments as possible for the next two weeks of school, or for the duration of the block of time for which schoolwork will be done.
3. Fill out sticky notes for the next two weeks of work for each subject, then place in the respective class column in the Planned Schoolwork section of the board. These are the students' assignments for the next two weeks and should correspond with the teacher's assignments for each subject.
4. Hold a daily Stand-up Meeting to select schoolwork (class assignments, tasks or smaller sub-tasks) from the Planned Schoolwork section and place them in the Today's Schoolwork section. This is a good time to encourage positive, collaborative, parent and student problem-solving. Together, the parent and student choose only the schoolwork that the student intends to complete for the current day. These are the student's commitments. This should result in a small group of tasks in the Today's Schoolwork section to be completed throughout that day.
5. Select the first task to be worked from Today's Schoolwork group of tasks and place the sticky note on the red and white target. This is the Target Task the student is to be physically working on <u>now</u>.
6. When the student completes the Target Task, they remove the sticky from the target and place it in the Finished Schoolwork section. These are the students' achievements.
7. If the student gets stuck or cannot proceed without help, then they either 1) write the issue on a sticky note, place it in the Desktop section and skip the item or 2) they place the Target Task in the Desktop then select the next task from the Today's Schoolwork group of tasks, place it on the target and begin work on that task. The Desktop items will be discussed as soon as possible or during the daily Stand-up Meeting.
8. The parent glances at *The Schoolwork Success System* board every few hours to check on the status of the work in progress.
9. The next day, return to step four.
10. At the end of the block period, return to step one.

2. Block Planning

The first step in the Schoolwork Success System is to conduct what we call schoolwork "block planning". A schoolwork block of time (or simply a "block") is defined as an *iterative, one to four-week period of time*. Ideally, the block is a duration of two weeks because teachers typically assign tasks with due dates beyond the current week. On the other hand, some teachers assign schoolwork weekly. As students get older, schoolwork often gets more complex, with due dates pushed further out. For example, studying for a test three weeks away or writing an essay due on the first of the next month. The concept is the block of time should reflect the average cadence or frequency at which schoolwork is assigned.

Figure 2 below illustrates the block period highlighted in blue. A typical block starts on a Monday and continues through the Friday of the second week. In Figure 2 the block period starts on May 4th and ends on May 15th. Over the duration of the block, the student concentrates their effort on completing all school assignments, or parts of assignments, planned to be completed within the block timeframe. Those assignments are either due during the block or must be worked on during the block timeframe to meet a due date beyond the block period. The block is iterative because The Schoolwork Success System starts over at the beginning of each block period. For example, for a two-week block there are two blocks in one month, and four blocks in two months. For the purposes of this handbook we will describe how a two-week block works.

Block Period

Monday	Tuesday	Wednesday	Thursday	Friday	No School	No School
4-May	5-May	6-May	7-May	8-May	9-May	10-May
Monday	Tuesday	Wednesday	Thursday	Friday	No School	No School
11-May	12-May	13-May	14-May	15-May	16-May	17-May

Figure 2

Block planning is a one-hour collaborative activity between the parent and student, to identify and record on sticky notes the work that will be accomplished over the next two weeks (the block). The meeting should take place either at the end of the tenth day, a Friday, or at the beginning of the first day of the block, a Monday morning. I have found that some teachers upload assignments over the weekend therefore Monday morning may be better. Block planning for a two-week block should take no longer than one hour. It may take longer the first few iterations, but after some practice, it should take less than an hour.

For the first block planning session, determine the start and finish dates for the block; then write those dates in the designated area at the top right corner [Figure 1, item 5] of The Schoolwork Success Board. Today's Date is updated during a short daily face-to-face meeting which will be discussed later.

Once the block period is known, obtain the next two weeks' school assignments for every subject from the teachers, an online student assignment portal, or a syllabus. The student and parent will use this information to jointly plan a two-week block of schoolwork, typically starting on a Monday and ending on the Friday after next. Write the start and finish dates in the upper right corner of the Task Board.

3.   Planned Schoolwork: My Assignments

Next, organize schoolwork tasks. To begin, select a sticky note color for each subject as shown in Figure 3 on page 11. For example, orange for social studies, blue for math, green for science, and yellow for language arts. The same color should not be used more than twice. If using just one color of sticky note, write the subject name or initials along with the assignment on the sticky note.

A sticky note represents a single schoolwork task. A task can be an entire assignment, part of an assignment, or small chunks of an assignment. In most cases, a schoolwork task will be the entire assignment. In other cases, a task may have several sub-tasks or steps. For example, a task written on a sticky note could represent multiple math problems, reading a chapter in a book, writing a first draft of an essay, or doing a science experiment. Each student has a different capacity for doing their work, and for different subjects or assignments. The size of the task on the sticky note should be roughly equivalent to their capability, and what they can get done during one study period.

A single schoolwork task is what the student can realistically accomplish in one study period. This is important for "right-sizing" the schoolwork to the unique capacity of the student. A study period is the length of time the student typically takes to get focused on a single task and concentrate for an uninterrupted period of time. A short break can be taken in between study periods. The average study period for one student may be 20-minutes, whereas another student may be comfortable with a one-hour study period, depending on the individual student's ability to focus and concentrate on a given task. Some tasks will be more difficult than others and require more time, while others, which may be of particular interest to the student may take up more time in a given study period.

Initially, the student will have the best insight into what they can get done in a study period. The parent should encourage them to guess how long it will take. Right-sizing the task on the sticky note takes practice, but as that experience is gained the parent and student will be able to more accurately estimate the time required for a task. Don't worry! It does not have to be perfect at first. You can adjust the priority and size of an assignment anytime during the schoolwork block. Remember: a schoolwork block is a two-week iteration of schooling.

For each subject in the "Planned Schoolwork" section of the board, write each individual schoolwork task (the full or partial schoolwork assignment) and the due date on a single sticky note that corresponds to the color of the subject, see Figure 3. It is best to have the student fill out the sticky notes to help them remember what needs to be done. Nothing more than the task description and due date should be written on the sticky note. The name or description of the assignment can be abbreviated. What's important is that the task and the dues date are understood by both parent and student. When done, place the sticky note in the respective "My Assignments" column.

Planned Schoolwork

My Assignments

Priority	Social Studies	Math	Science	Language Arts	Music	Class or Meetings
1	Due 5/6 Read Ch.3 Questions 1-4	Due 5/6 Lesson 12 Prob 1-6	Due 5/15 Purify Water Step 1: Materials	Due 5/6 Bio Essay 1st Draft		Science Tuesday 1-3pm
2	Due 5/11 Read Ch.4 Q: 1-4	Due 5/8 Lesson 12 Prob 7-12	Due 5/15 Purify Water Step 2: Conduct Experiment	Due 5/15 Bio Essay 2nd Draft		Math Wednesday 2-3pm
3	Due 5/16 Read Ch.5 Q: 1-4	Due 5/13 Lesson 13 Prob 1-5	Due 5/15 Purify H_2O Step 3: Observe	Due 5/20 Bio Essay Final Draft		Math Monday 2-3pm
4		Due 5/15 Lesson 13 Prob 6-10	Due 5/15 Purify H_2O Step 4: Draft Report			Lang Arts Tuesday 10-11am Lang Arts

Figure 3

If the assignment is larger than usual or will last for several weeks, such as a big science experiment, then it should be broken down into several smaller, more manageable chunks or sub-tasks such as: 1) collect materials 2) set up experiment 3) conduct experiment and take notes 4) write report. Each sub-task would become a single task therefore a separate sticky note would be written for each sub-task along with the due date. See the science column in Figure 3.

As each sticky note is written, the student should place the sticky note under the respective Planned Schoolwork subject column, <u>in the order of priority</u>. This is a good opportunity for the parent and student to collaborate. The order of priority is usually dictated by the due date.

4.   Final Planning Review

Once all the assignments for the next two weeks are placed on the board in the order of their priority, the student and parent will have a visual representation of the next two weeks' worth of schoolwork. There should be no more shuffling through syllabi, clicking on links at the last minute to figure out the next few assignments, or searching for what assignments are late, or emailing teachers for progress reports. It's now all laid out in an organized, colorful, visual format for parent and student to obtain the most important information at-a-glance.

Now it is time for the parent and student to do a final review. Make sure that the sticky notes are in the correct order of priority, sequence of work and broken down into realistic-sized tasks tailored to the capability of the individual student. Again, this is a great opportunity for the parent and student to spend an hour every two weeks focused on how the schoolwork is progressing.

If each sticky note is in the correct order of priority and a reasonable amount of work is written on the sticky note, leave it "as is." This will likely be the majority of the sticky notes. If not, then have a conversation with your student to revise the amount of work written on the sticky. For example, assume there is a reading assignment with six essay questions. The student believes they are capable of reading the entire essay and answering the first two questions in about 30-minutes, which is the duration of their typical study period without taking a break. The student believes they can answer the remaining four questions during a second study period. In this case, there will now be two yellow sticky notes: one for reading the essay and answering questions 1 and 2; and another sticky note for answering questions 3, 4, 5 and 6. Another example would be a math assignment with 20 problems. The student and parent agree that it should take about two hours to do the full assignment. They know this because the last two math assignments each took about two hours. Let's say the student believes they can complete 10 problems in a one-hour study period. In this case, there would be two green sticky notes: one for problems 1-10 and the other for problems 11-20, respectively.

Again, right-sizing the task written on the sticky note is very important and takes some time to master, because each student has a different capacity for schoolwork and the ability to focus. *The Schoolwork Success System* is designed for success, but if we assign tasks that are too big, or beyond the student's capability, we could be setting them up for failure. The system is a tool for both the parent and student to learn how to right-size tasks or sub-tasks as well as to identify, as early as possible, where the student needs help. When tasks are not getting done, the parent asks either the student or teacher why? Asking "why" is part of the system. The intent is for the parent and student to work together in a positive way to determine the cause of delays, missing assignments or poor performance, and then find solutions. When parents have to wait until parent-teacher conferences or report cards to learn about the impediments or challenges to the students' progress, the student is likely already falling behind and their schoolwork piling up, which is overwhelming and demoralizing for the student. With *The Schoolwork Success System*, the parent and student work together to make estimates about what work can be done in a given study period. After just a couple of two-week schoolwork blocks both the parent and student should have a better understanding of the student's capability and capacity, as well as their strengths and weaknesses.

The two-week block planning is now complete. With all assignments for the next two-weeks written on sticky notes and placed in order of priority in the appropriate column, we are almost ready to begin a two-week block. First, we need to provide clarity and boundaries for the conduct of the schoolwork.

5.   System Rules

"Rules" are an important element of *The Schoolwork Success System*. The lower left area of the board is dedicated to the rules that make the system work best. Rules are made at the discretion of the parent but with input from the student. Developing rules is an excellent opportunity for the parent and student to make positive, collaborative decisions resulting in greater buy-in and reduced conflict. For example, Alan found that sometimes it was more productive to focus on the same subject all day long because of the learning curve. We realized that as Alan became more familiar with a given textbook, he was able to flip through it faster resulting in completing work faster and more accurately. He also realized that he would build on his learning better when ideas from a previous lesson were fresh on his mind making him more productive. Another rule we used was never to spend more than 10 minutes on a given math problem. Too often he was spending 30 or more minutes on a single problem which cut into his time to do his other assignments. Rules should provide unquestionable clarity for the student and alignment among parent, student and the school. There should not be many rules, just the most important ones that enable the smooth, productive flow of schoolwork. Typical rules are:

- When are break times?
- How long is the schoolwork day?
- How should the tasks be prioritized or approved?
- Who verifies or approves the completed schoolwork?
- What are the requirements or criteria for tasks to be declared done?
- Will the student work on a variety of subjects throughout the day or focus on several tasks for one subject?
- Under what conditions is the Target Task to be moved from the target to the Finished Schoolwork column?
- Does Dad need to review my assignment for correctness and completeness or can the student make that decision on her own?

The rules should reflect boundaries for the workflow, address behavioral nuances and influence corrective actions. For purposes of getting your student's buy-in on the rules, I recommend developing rules in a positive, collaborative way between parent and student.

6.   Today's Schoolwork: My Commitments

To kick-off the first day of the block period, the parent and student must hold a Stand-up Meeting to select which sticky notes will be selected from the Planned Schoolwork section and placed in the "Today's Schoolwork" section. These selected schoolwork tasks are the tasks the student commits to completing by the end of the given day. This activity of selecting and removing the schoolwork items from the Planned Schoolwork section and then placing them in the Today's Schoolwork section is a daily ritual conducted during the Stand-up Meeting.

7.   The Morning Stand-up Meeting

Typically, a block of schoolwork starts on a Monday. Each and every day, beginning on the first morning of the block, the parent and student stand in front of *The Schoolwork Success System* (S3) board and hold a brief "Stand-up Meeting." The purpose of the Stand-up Meeting is to update the S3 board and discover any issues delaying or interfering with progress.

Why do we call it a Stand-up Meeting? Because the student and parent will literally stand in front of the board and have a clear, concise conversation about the status of the board. A study from the Texas A&M Health Science Center School of Public Health showed that people often think better on their feet. Also, standing is shown to motivate participants to finish quickly so that they can sit down sooner. The daily parent-student Stand-up Meeting should be a timed meeting that lasts no longer than 15 minutes. The Stand-up Meeting is a scripted meeting that asks only these same three questions, each day:

What was completed yesterday?

Asking this question provides both the parent and student time to briefly reflect and gain insight into the previous day's progress. When asking the question, the parent and student refer to the Today's Schoolwork and Finished Schoolwork columns. This fun and rewarding activity motivate students because they are able to see in near-real time their incremental achievements. Watching the Finished Schoolwork column grow is nearly immediate gratification which is inspiring for most students. This is also the time to praise or reward the student for their progress. For the parent, they are able to visually see the students' progress, hold the student accountable for their progress or lack thereof, identify their strength and weaknesses, and expose any areas that are challenging or not getting completed in a timely manner. It is an opportunity to spot patterns and gain insight into the students' capabilities and challenges. If one of yesterday's tasks is incomplete then it can either remain in Today's Schoolwork or it could be returned to the Planned Schoolwork section and reprioritized. What's most important is we discover the issue early and ask "why" the task did not get done?

What can be realistically completed today?

Each day, the parent and student select new tasks from the Planned Schoolwork column and place them in the Today's Schoolwork column as the students' commitment for the day. This is also the time to make any changes or adjustments to the plan. For example, the teacher may ask for a revised essay that is due in two days. The parent, acting as a trusted advisor or coach, can help the student determine what they are capable to doing during the day. The parent helps the student determine what is most important given the due dates, the amount of work remaining, and any other factors that may impact the student's ability to complete the work – such as a task being too big to be done in one day. In that case, the student and parent may decide to breakdown the assignments into smaller tasks. At this time the student makes a commitment to accomplishing the days' schoolwork tasks.

What areas do you need help with?

When the student needs help with an assignment it creates a barrier to progress. Asking this question helps make the parent aware of the students' challenges at the earliest possible moment. When asking this question, refer to the "Desktop" column of the board (more to come on the Desktop). How many times did you learn at the end of the term or from a report card that your student was struggling with a certain subject? By discovering this at the earliest possible time, we can encourage the student to reach out to the teacher, opt to intervene to facilitate the students' learning, or coordinate with the school or teacher to obtain support on behalf of your student.

After the few sticky notes selected for the days' schoolwork are taken from the Planned Schoolwork column and placed in the Today's Schoolwork column, there should be a small grouping of sticky notes under the words My Commitment. The parent and student should then reorder those sticky notes, prioritizing from top to bottom, which tasks will be done during that specific day. The intention is that the student completes all tasks in the group of sticky notes by the end of the day. This 15-minute meeting occurs every morning at the start of the day.

If the student did not complete all the previous days' Today's Schoolwork tasks, then during the Stand-Up Meeting you can choose whether to return the incomplete task to the Planned Schoolwork section to be reprioritized or done at a different time; or it can remain in the Today's Schoolwork section as a top priority. The most important aspect of incomplete tasks is for the student and parent to understand *why* the task was incomplete. Was it too big? Too difficult? Or, did the student get distracted? Then find a remedy for the issue.

8.   The Target Task

Notice again in the Today's Schoolwork column there is a red and white Target towards the bottom of the column. This is the "Target Task". The purpose of the Target Task is to have a specified location for the task-at-hand so there is no question what the student should be doing. The task in front of the student should be the one that is being worked on.

The Target Task is selected from the Today's Schoolwork group of sticky notes (today's tasks) and sticking it to the center of the target. This provides clarity and alignment between the student and parent about what is supposed to be working on <u>now</u>. It also acts as a reminder to the student not to switch tasks and stay focused only on the Target until complete. When the task in the target is done according to the rules (more on rules below) then the sticky can be removed from the target and placed in the Finished Schoolwork column. At this point, the process is repeated. The next task to be worked is removed from the group of sticky notes in the Today's Schoolwork column and placed in the Target for the student to begin work on. This flow of schoolwork is continued each day, 5 days per week for two weeks (a two-week iteration or block of schoolwork). In a very short time, the parent and student will develop a rhythm of planning and completing schoolwork, while at the same time, identifying areas in which the student may need support.

The main idea is to regulate the flow of schoolwork for the student and parent alike to remain situationally aware of the schoolwork that is being done or is partially done. This helps reduce the chances of missing an assignment, partially completing an assignment or forgetting to turn-in an assignment. When this does happen, assignments pile up on the student causing a bottleneck to producing completed assignments. Maintaining awareness and control of the completion of assignments can reduce a lot of anxiety, stress and conflict.

Notice that under the target symbol is an area of white space. This space is for any notes related to the day's work or the Target. For example, how long to work on the given target task, or what time the day finishes, e.g., 3:30 pm. Whatever is written below the target is at the parent's discretion, and it should relate to the given day's schoolwork.

9.   The Desktop

So, what happens when the student is stuck, is confused or needs help? First, the parent and student should establish a rule for this situation. The rule could be "Ask mom first." If mom can't help, the student may stop work, remove the sticky note from the target, and place it in the "Desktop" area at the bottom right corner of the board. Then, accordioning to the rules, maybe she sends an Instant Message (IM) to the teacher. The purpose of the Desktop section is to have a place to identify and track important items or issues that are causing schoolwork delays or challenges. When the parent glances at the board throughout the day and sees an item in the Desktop area, it is a visual signal to the parent that there is an issue. This helps to quickly identify areas that are impeding the students' progress and where support is needed most. Additionally, it prevents the student from spending too much time on one item resulting in having burned up critical time, better spent on other committed tasks for which they are proficient. The Desktop sets aside, or isolates, the difficult item for follow-up so the student can carry-on with other tasks and make better daily progress. The Desktop can also be used to simply record on a sticky note a question the student or parent may have for follow-up with the teacher.

No longer does the parent need to wait for parent-teacher conferences or report cards to identify problem areas or hear about work that is not getting done. The Desktop is a function to discover and address those challenges at the earliest possible moment. To resolve Desktop items the parent may provide support, the parent may ask the student to reach out to the teacher, or the parent could email or call the teacher to ask for assistance. The principle is having a place where issues are identified and stored for immediate or short-term follow-up to reduce the possibility of the student falling behind or not getting support due to a lack of parental or teacher awareness.

10.   Finished Schoolwork: My Achievements

When Today's Schoolwork tasks are completed, they should be reviewed at some point by the parent. Not necessarily for correctness but, at a minimum, for completeness. This can be done immediately after the work is completed, <u>before</u> moving the Target Task to the "Finished Schoolwork" area; or the student can move the Target Task to the Finished Schoolwork area, for the parent to check it for completion at a later time. Occasionally, students forget to turn-in an assignment or can't remember if they completed a task. The Finished Schoolwork area helps parents and students keep track of weekly achievements. A quick check during the Stand-up meeting may be sufficient. It all depends on what your student needs to facilitate the process. What is important is a quick check-in during the day to verify the task is 100% complete. This is also a good time to check the Desktop for any unfinished work or issues which need attention.

11.   Repeat the Process

The Schoolwork Success System is an iterative process – repeating over and over. At the end of the two-week block period, the parent and student spend an hour reviewing upcoming assignments, breaking down large tasks and doing block planning for the next two weeks. When block planning is finished the two-week iteration starts all over. The parent and student go back to a routine of holding daily Stand-up Meetings, selecting assignments for Today's Schoolwork, doing those assignments in a prioritized manner, and placing the completed tasks in the Finished Schoolwork section. When the student encounters a roadblock, they write it down on a sticky note and place it in the Desktop for follow-up. This continues until the end of the two-week block period, then repeat.

12.   The Schoolwork Success System in Action – An Example

In the following example, we walk through the first two days of a 10-day block period. The setting is a typical two days of schoolwork for Alan, with the schoolwork tasks flowing from the Planned Schoolwork area through the Today's Schoolwork and Target, then ending in the Finished Schoolwork area. The Desktop is also used when an issue or impediment arises.

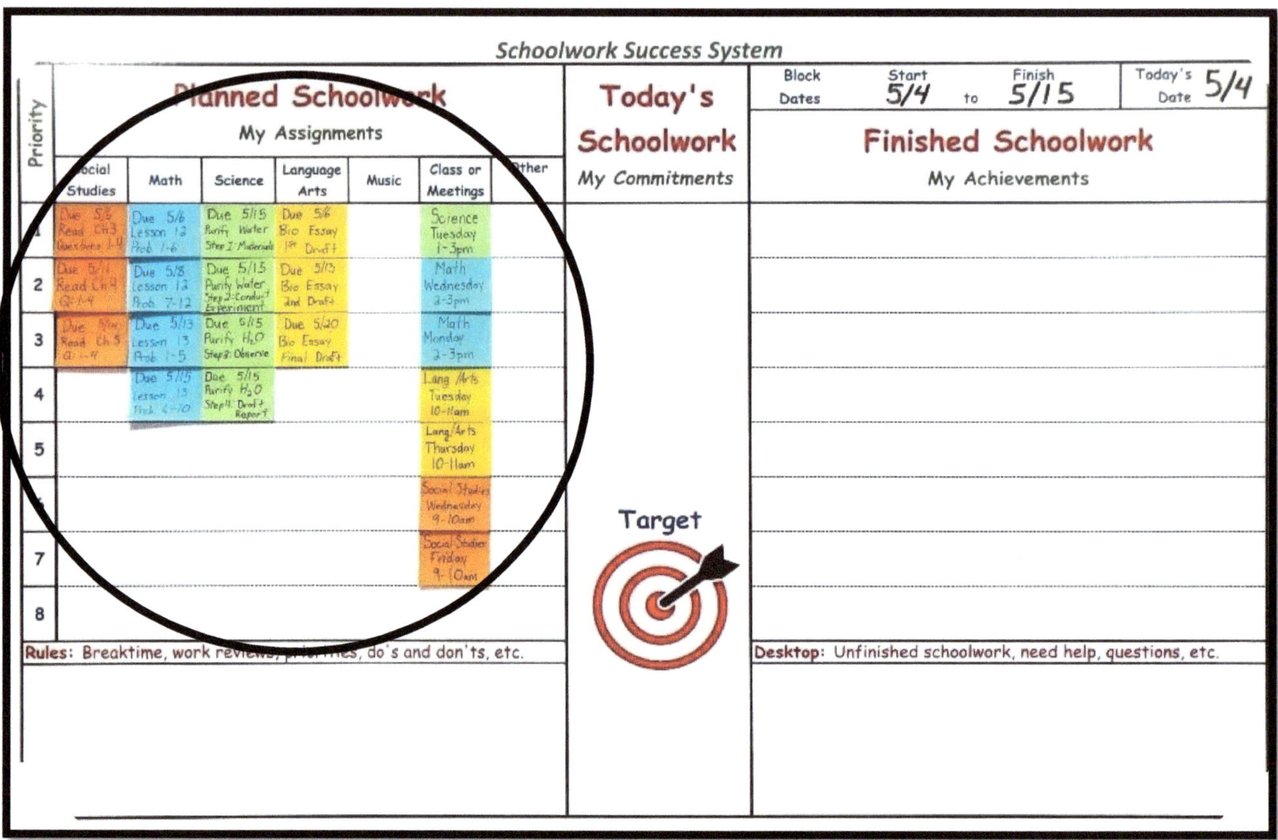

Figure 4

Day 1:

On the first day of the block period the first thing that is accomplished is block planning. As can be seen in the above Figure 4, the next two weeks of Alan's assignments are written in simple terms on sticky notes then placed in the Planned Schoolwork area in the corresponding subject column. In this example, orange sticky notes represent Social Studies tasks, blue sticky notes represent Math tasks, Green for Science tasks, and yellow for Language Arts tasks. The block period dates are written in the top right-hand corner. The dates for this block period are May 4th to May 15th. Today's date is May 4th.

For the majority of the subjects, the order of priority is dictated by the due date which is written on the sticky note. However, for science we have the same due date for all tasks but we have four separate steps therefore the order of priority is based on the sequence of steps.

The tasks in the "Class or Meetings" column are for reoccurring classes or one-time only meetings. There may be online classes scheduled at the same time each week, say a Tuesday and Thursday. To ensure the student is aware of the class, create a sticky note with a class description, the date and time for each class then reuse the sticky note. In other words, on the day of the class move the respective sticky note from the Planned Schoolwork section and place it in the Today's Schoolwork column. When the class is over, instead of placing the sticky note in the Finished Schoolwork column return it to the Planned Schoolwork "Class or Meeting" column so it can be reused.

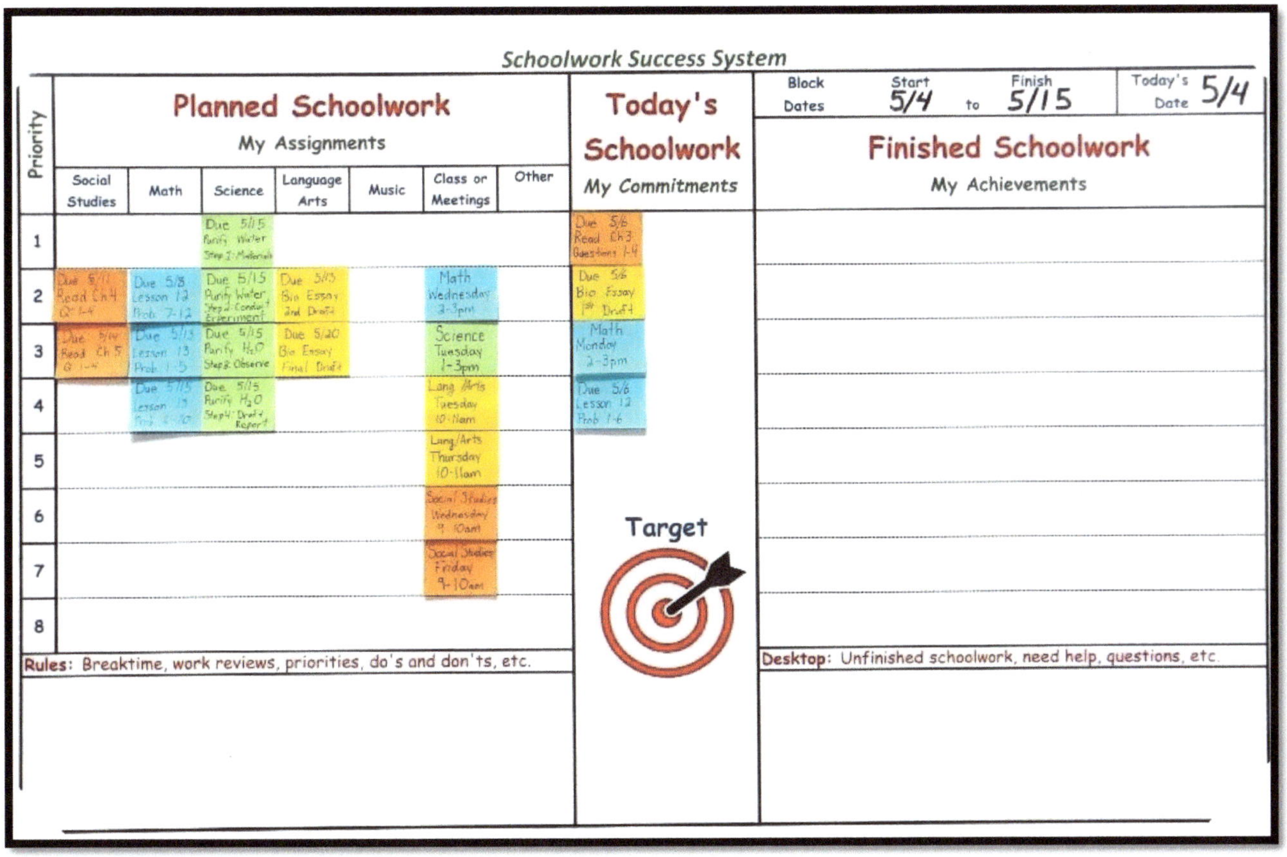

Schoolwork Success System

Block Dates — Start **5/4** to Finish **5/15** — Today's Date **5/4**

Planned Schoolwork — My Assignments

Priority	Social Studies	Math	Science	Language Arts	Music	Class or Meetings	Other
1			Due 5/15 Purify Water Step 1 Materials				
2	Due 5/11 Read Ch 4 Q 1-4	Due 5/8 Lesson 12 Prob 7-12	Due 5/15 Purify Water Step 3 Conduct Experiment	Due 5/13 Bio Essay 2nd Draft		Math Wednesday 2-3pm	
3	Due 5/14 Read Ch 5 Q 1-4	Due 5/13 Lesson 13 Prob 1-5	Due 5/15 Purify H₂O Step 2 Observe	Due 5/20 Bio Essay Final Draft		Science Tuesday 1-3pm	
4		Due 5/15 Lesson 13 Prob 6-10	Due 5/15 Purify H₂O Step 4 Draft Report			Lang Arts Tuesday 10-11am	
5						Lang/Arts Thursday 10-11am	
6						Social Studies Wednesday 9-10am	
7						Social Studies Friday 9-10am	
8							

Rules: Breaktime, work reviews, priorities, do's and don'ts, etc.

Today's Schoolwork — My Commitments

- Due 5/6 Read Ch 3 Questions 1-4
- Due 5/6 Bio Essay 1st Draft
- Math Monday 2-3pm
- Due 5/6 Lesson 12 Prob 1-6

Target

Finished Schoolwork — My Achievements

Desktop: Unfinished schoolwork, need help, questions, etc.

Figure 5

After block planning is complete, we select the tasks that will be done for the day and remove them from the Planned Schoolwork area and place them in the Today's Schoolwork column. In this case we chose one Social Studies task, one Language Arts task, a Math task and a 2:00 pm re-occurring Math class task. For the example, Alan has a re-occurring Math class every Monday and Wednesday from 2:00 to 3:00 pm. The result is a group of tasks that Alan will commit to completing by the end of the day.

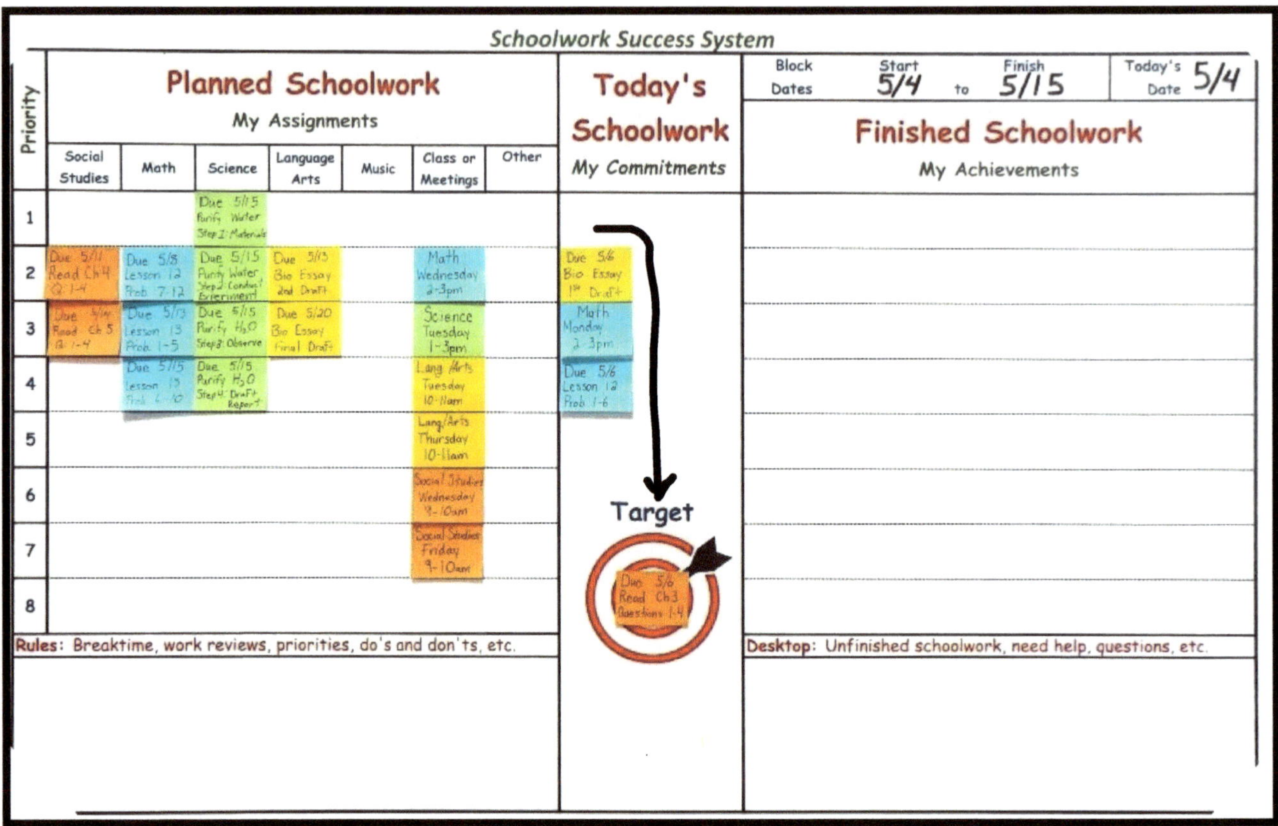

Figure 6

The next step is to select the Target Task – the task that Alan will work on now. We pull the Target Task from the Today's Schoolwork group of tasks and place it in the middle of the red and white target. In this case it is an orange Social Studies sticky that reads "Read Ch. 3 and [answer] questions 1-4". With the sticky note in the target area, there is no question about what Alan should be working on now. This will be his only focus for the next study period, typically about an hour or so.

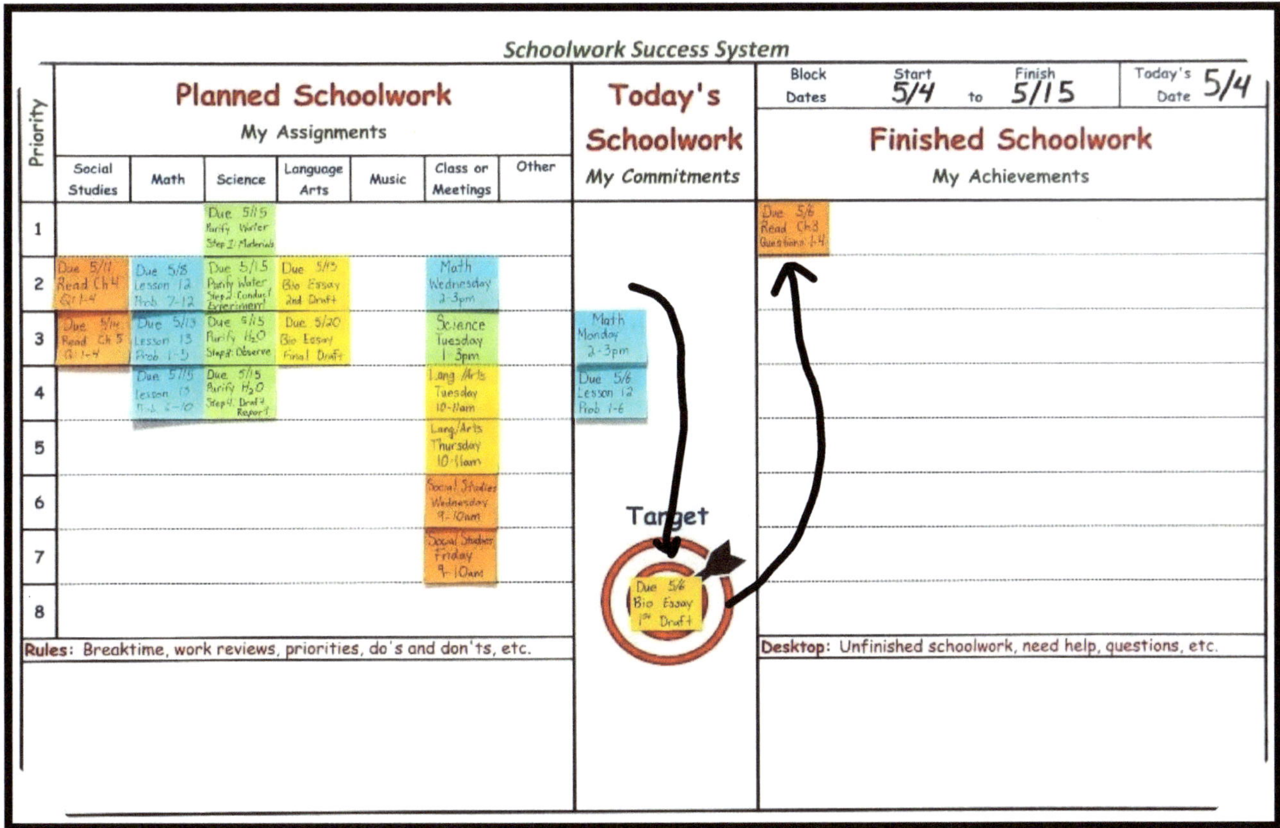

Figure 7

Once the Social Studies Target Task is complete it is removed from the target area and placed into the Finished Schoolwork area. It is best if the parent can check the students work before moving the Target Task into the Finished Schoolwork area but sometimes this is not always convenient or verification can be done at a different time such as immediately following the morning Stand-up meeting.

After moving the completed Target Task to the Finished Schoolwork area we select the next task from the above group of committed tasks (Today's Schoolwork), place the sticky on the red and white target and then commence working on the Target Task until complete. In this situation the yellow Language Arts task is the next Target Task. The workflow continues at this cadence throughout the day.

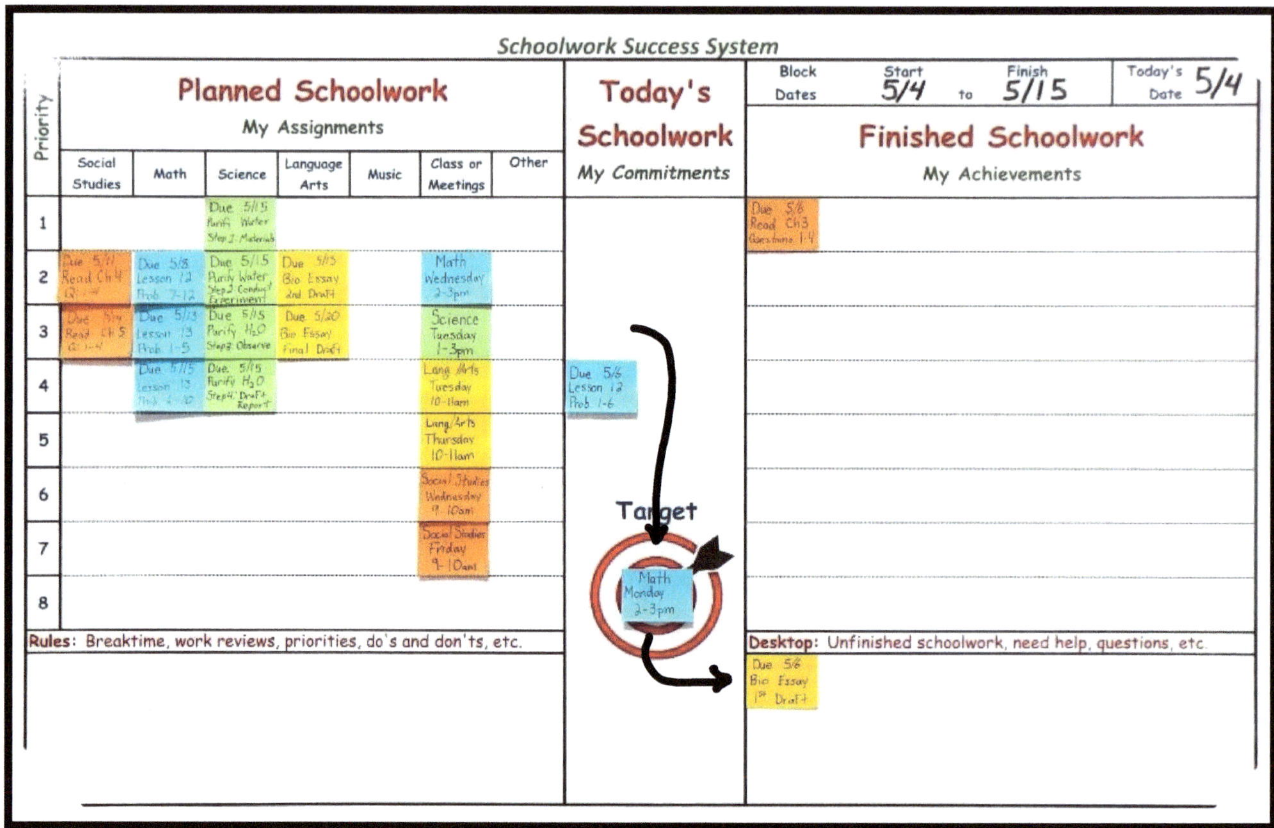

Figure 8

While working on the yellow Language Arts Target Task Alan runs into a problem. The Target Task is to write a first draft of a biographical essay. He wrote his ideas down about some of the key events in his life but he is not sure how to structure the timeline of his essay. So, after 10 minutes of struggling with this part of the essay he stops work, removes the Target Task sticky note from the target and places it in the Desktop area for follow-up later with either me or his teacher. A sticky note in the Desktop is a signal that something needs attention!

At this point, Alan has two remaining schoolwork tasks for the day. He has a 2:00 pm online Math class and Math Lesson 12, problems 1-6 to complete. Since it is now about 12:30 pm Alan breaks for lunch then gets ready for his 2:00 pm class. He decides not to start on Lesson 12 because this will be part of the 2:00 pm class.

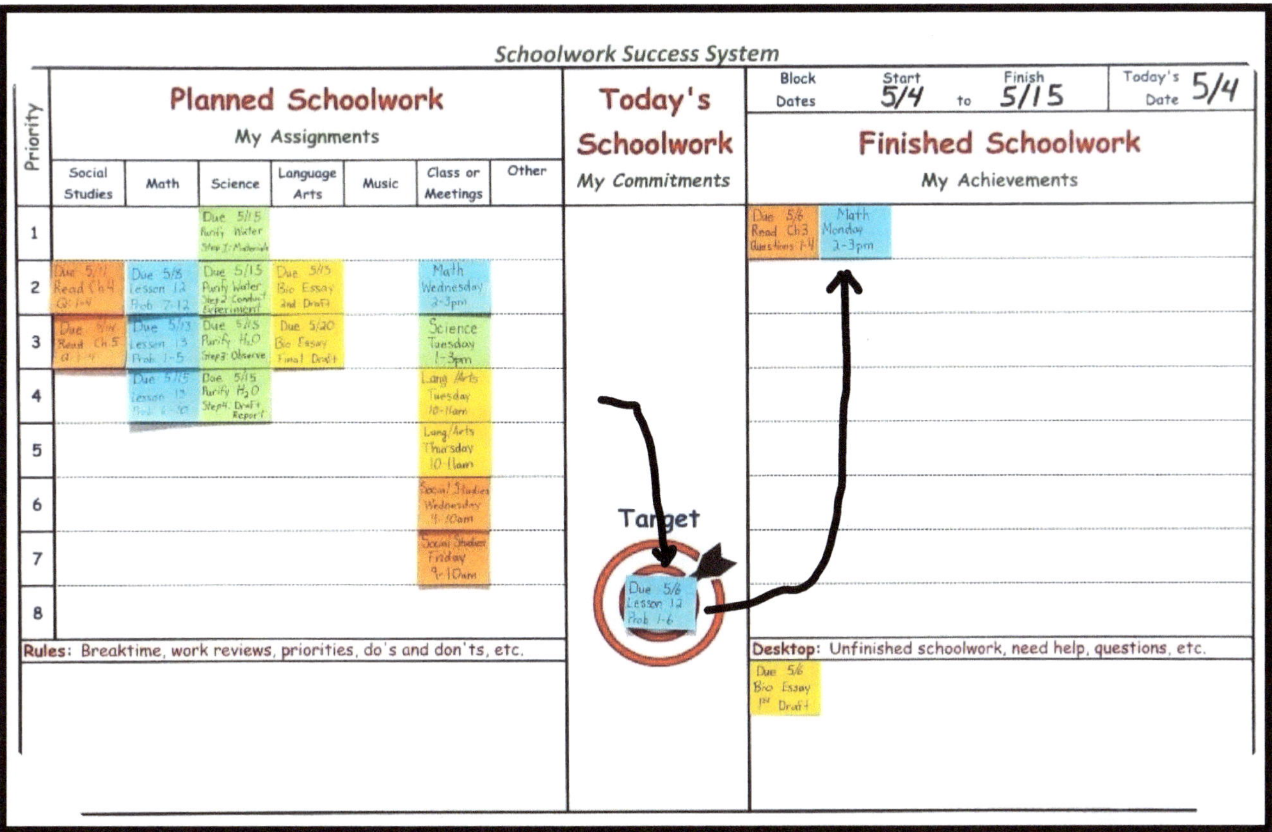

Figure 9

After the 2:00 pm Math class is finished Alan feels better prepared to do Math Lesson 12, problems 1-6 therefore he moves the blue Math 2:00 online class sticky note to the Finished Schoolwork area and then moves the last remaining blue Math task Lesson 12, problems 1-6 to the target area. This becomes the final Target Task to be completed by the end of the day.

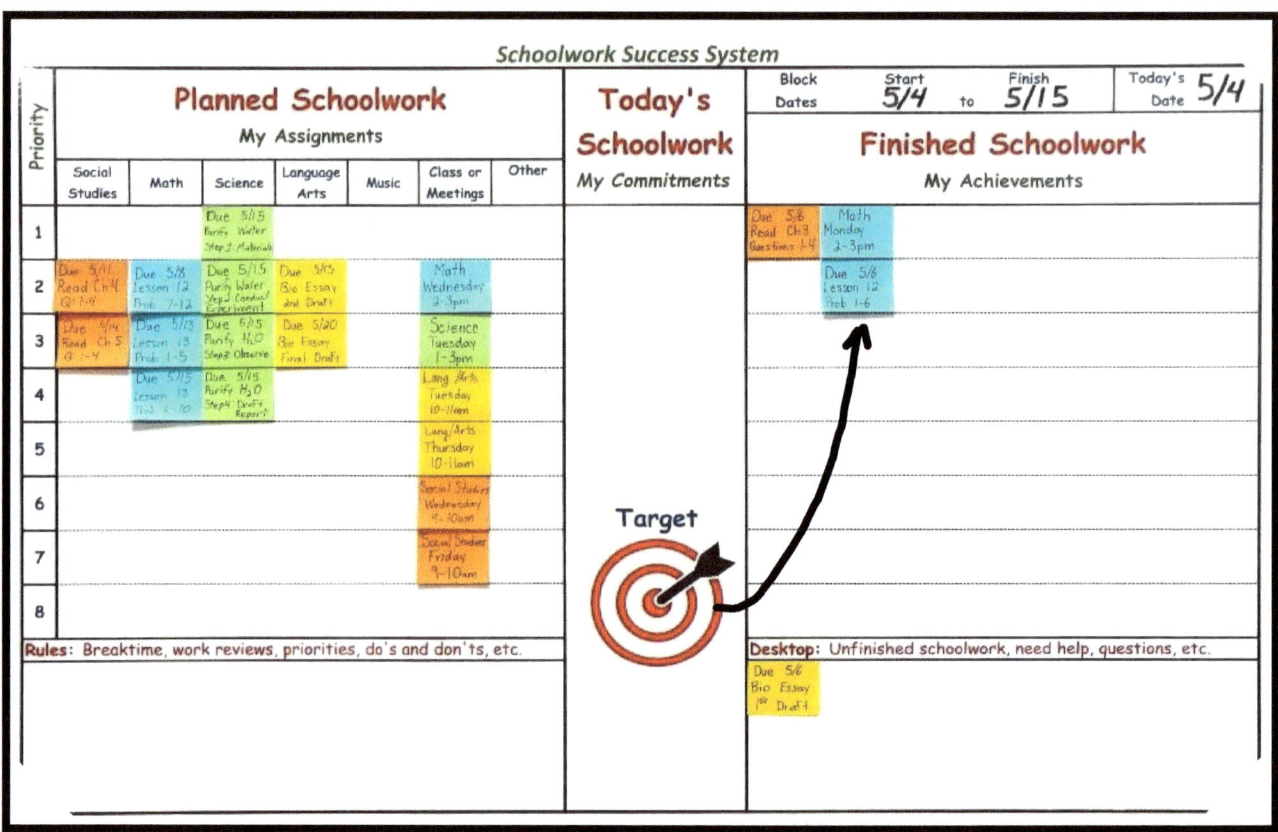

Figure 10

Once the last Target Task is complete, the day is over. All tasks were complete but for the first draft of the biographical essay, which can be found in the Desktop area. At the end of the day, the Today's Schoolwork area is now void of tasks, as it should be.

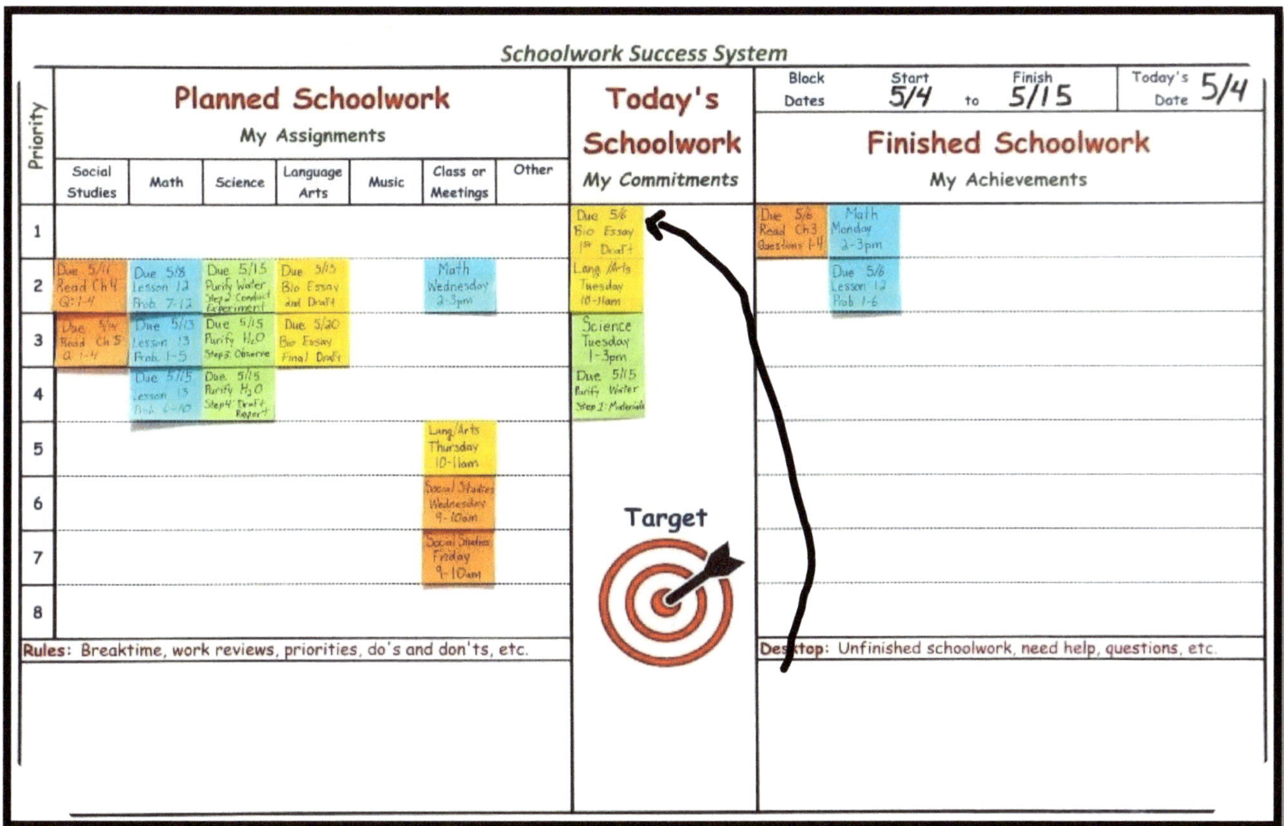

Figure 11

Day 2:

Today is Tuesday morning. The first thing that happens is Alan and I meet in front of the Schoolwork Success System board to hold a Stand-up meeting. One of us changes the date in the top right-hand corner of the board. We then review the Finished Schoolwork are and briefly discuss what was accomplished yesterday. I give him a pat on the back and ask him to continue the hard work. Additionally, Alan explains he had an issue with the timeline for his biographical essay. Fortunately, I could answer his question. If I could not, I would advise him to email his teacher today, and we would have filled out a sticky note for the Today's Schoolwork group.

The next thing we do is select the tasks that Alan will work on today. I typically ask Alan to select the tasks and physically remove them from the Planned Schoolwork area and place them in the Today's Schoolwork column. This way he touches and reads the sticky notes so that he gets familiar with the days' tasks and sets his mind on the work. I have found that there is better result when he makes the decisions.

For this particular day, Alan first moves the yellow sticky note from the Desktop back into the Today's Schoolwork column because I was able to answer his question, and he aims to finish the task today. Next, he selects the yellow "L/A Tuesday, 10:00-11:00 am online class" sticky and two science task stickys: "Science Tuesday, 1:00-3:00 pm" for an online class, and "Science Step 1: Materials" to be his daily commitments.

There are times when I ask Alan to explain his reasoning for choosing a particular task for today's schoolwork. He often has a good reason, but at other times I strongly suggest he select a different, more urgent task. We are careful not to select too much work, or too little work. We want to right-size his workload so that there is a high probability he will complete the day's schoolwork. The more we estimated his capability the more accurate we became, which resulted in greater confidence and much better productivity.

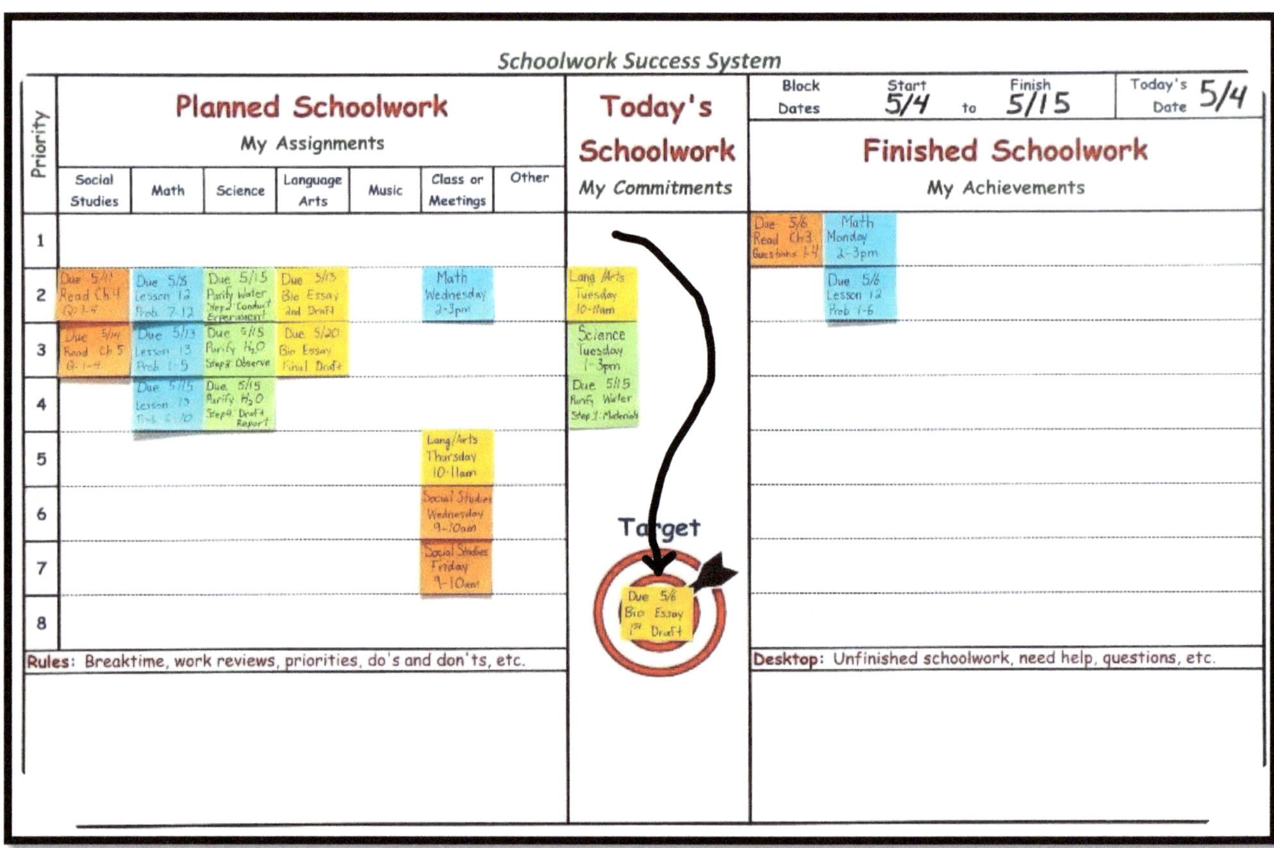

Figure 12

In figure 12, we are now finished with the daily Stand-up meeting and Alan is ready to begin today's schoolwork. His first Target Task is finishing the first draft of his biographical essay (the yellow Language Arts sticky note at the top of the Today's Schoolwork group of tasks).

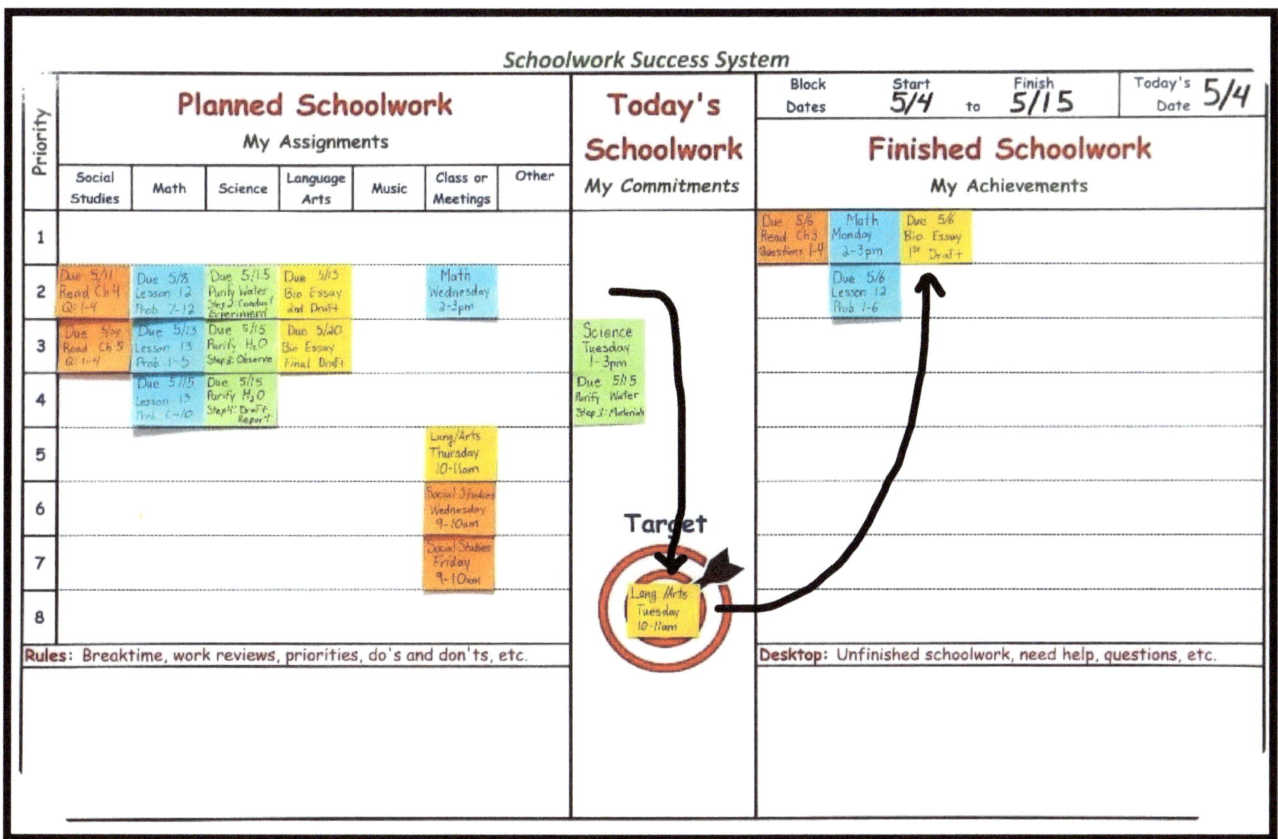

Figure 13

Once Alan completes the first draft of the biographical essay, he is ready for the next task. Alan removes the completed Target task from the red and white target and places it in the Finished Schoolwork area. Next, he pulls the next Target Task down from Today's Schoolwork group of tasks and places it on the target. In this case, he has a 10:00 am online class to attend. This workflow continues for the remainder of the day.

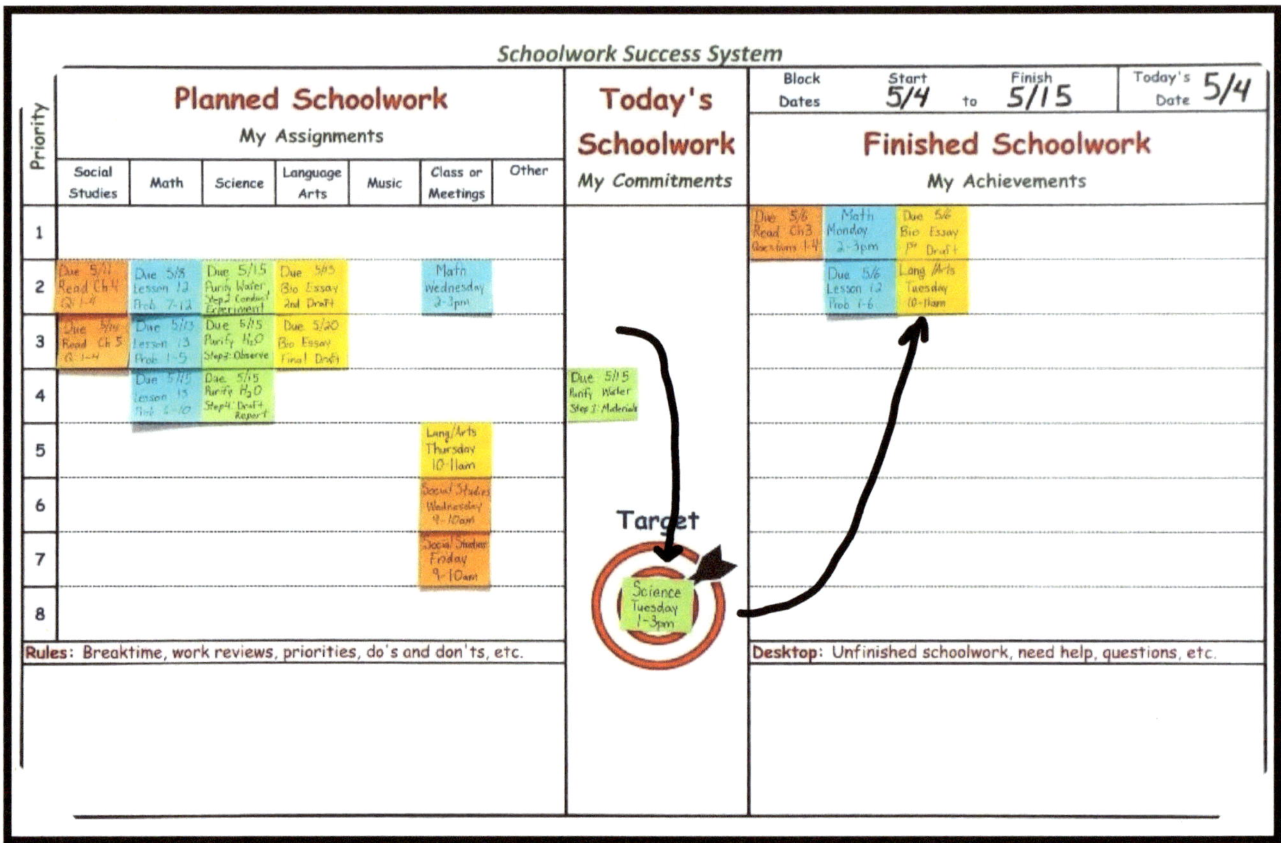

Figure 14

After Alan completes the online Language Arts class, he removes the yellow sticky from the target and places it in the Finished Schoolwork area. Next, he selects the top green sticky note from the remaining two sticky notes in the Today's Schoolwork group and places it on the target. This next task just happens to be a 1:00 pm online Science class he must attend. Since his online Language Arts class ended at 11:00 am and the next class does not start until 1:00 pm, Alan has some time to have lunch and get organized or do other school related tasks.

Note to the parent. It's very, very helpful to glance at the board occasionally to "spot check" the students work. Ask them "How's it going"? Or "Do you need any help"? I also ask Alan to briefly explain what he is working on, and "When will you be done?" The point is that it can be inspiring to the student for the parent to show genuine interest in their daily work, and also offer some help when possible. And, of course, we want to make sure the student is following *The Schoolwork Success System* process and making progress towards getting Today's Schoolwork accomplished.

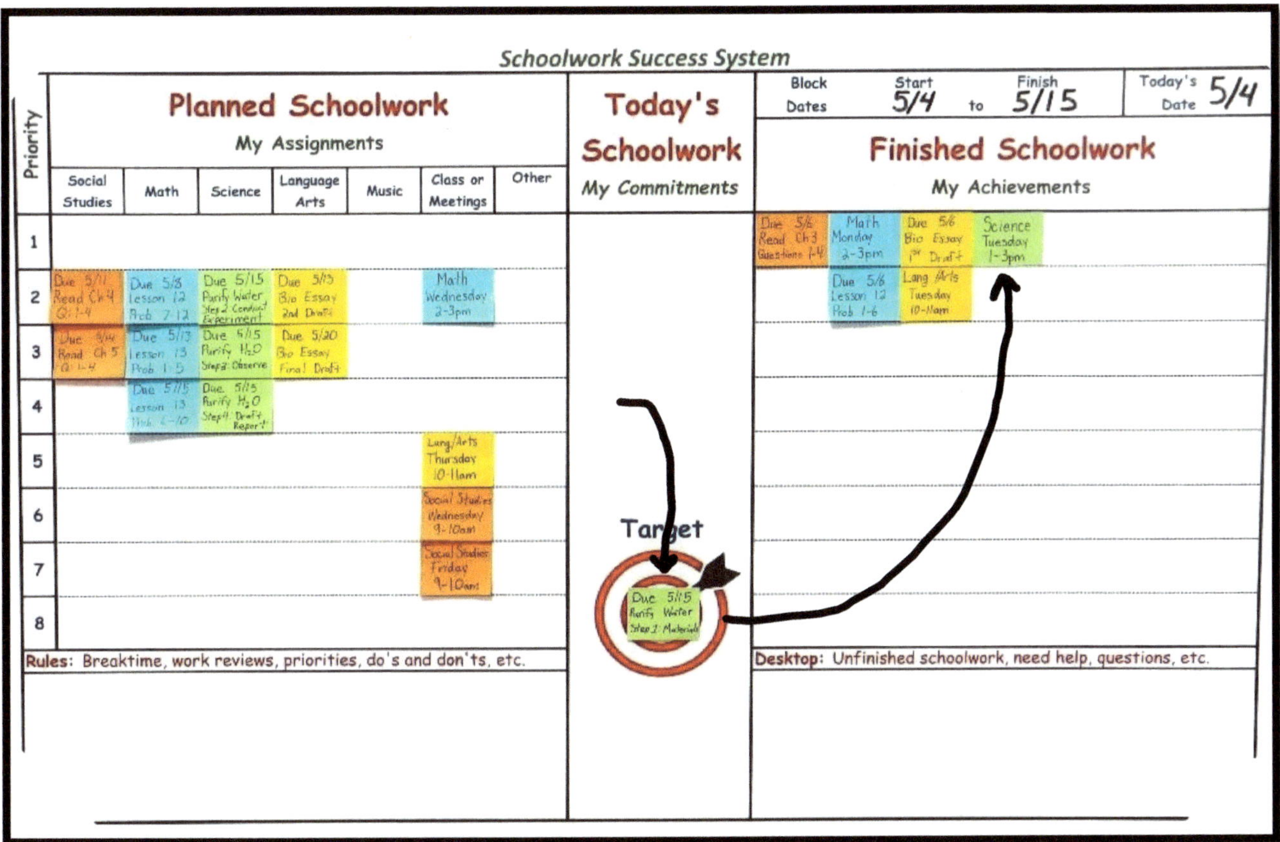

Figure 15

It's now 3:00 pm and Alan has just completed a 2-hour online science class. During the science class, the teacher explained to the student what was expected for the water purification home science project. There is now one sticky remaining in the Today's Schoolwork group of tasks. The next step is to remove the online Science class sticky note from the target and place it in the Finished Schoolwork area to continue to group Alan's schoolwork achievements. Once this is done, there is one last remaining green sticky note from the group of Today's Schoolwork. The task is Purify Water, Step 1: Materials. Alan places the remaining sticky on the target and then begins collecting household materials for his project.

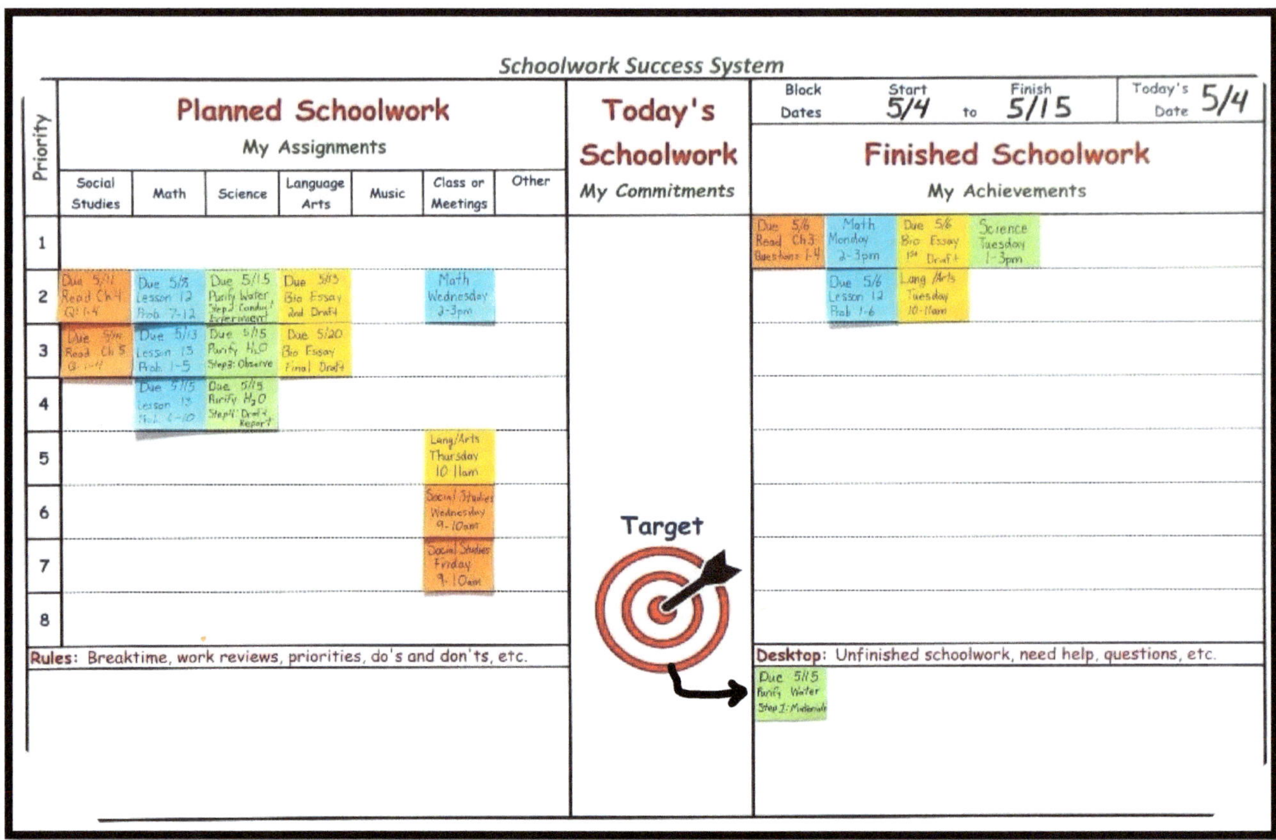

Figure 16

While Alan is collecting household materials, he realizes we are out of coffee filters (one of the items on the materials list). He wants to ask the teacher if he can use a piece of tightly woven cloth instead of the coffee filter. After collecting as many materials as possible, he stops doing his schoolwork task. Alan then removes the sticky note from the target and places it in the Desktop area as a reminder to follow-up with the teacher and to collect the remainder of the science project supplies. This end the 2nd day of the schoolwork block period.

As described in this example, the system continues until the last day of the block, typically on a Friday. At that time all sticky notes should be in the Finished Schoolwork area. This is a good time to celebrate the student's success or perhaps reward them with something that inspires them. On the Monday following the last day of the block, the parent and student repeat another 1-hour block planning session and then the block iteration starts over again. It is very helpful if the student gets an early start on writing assignments on sticky notes. Alan would do this in his free time during the day when he would finish an assignment early or immediately upon receiving a new assignment. The main idea is to develop and maintain the schoolwork flow in a cadence that is comfortable for the student while accomplishing the planned tasks in a predictable, prioritized manner as well as identifying potential roadblocks to progress so that they can be addressed at the earliest possible time.

10 Tips for Schoolwork Success

1. **Believe in the System**: Practice the procedures as described in this book. Modify and adjust the system to fit your particular parenting style and student needs while holding true to the basic principles of the Schoolwork Success System.

2. **Set up a dedicated Schoolwork Spot**: Make sure your student has a well-lit place to complete homework. Keep all school supplies easily accessible. Place the S3 Board in a location free of clutter, accessible and visible to the student, and in the same spot each day.

3. **Keep distractions to a minimum**: TV, loud music and cell phones can all be significant distractions.

4. **Help create a Daily Schedule**: Students work best at differing times, some in the morning, some in the afternoon and others may prefer to wait until after dinner.

5. **Use the Schoolwork Success System as your Plan**: The system uses what we know about adolescent brain development to breakdown the calendar, worktimes and assignments into manageable chunks.

6. **Get to know your child's teacher(s)**: Attend school events, such as parent-teacher conferences, to meet your child's teachers. Periodically check the teacher's website. Email the teacher for updates and suggestions. Ask about their homework policies and how you should be involved.

7. **Be your child's motivator**: Ask about assignments, projects, and tests. Encourage your student, check their work and offer suggestions. Be there for their questions and concerns. Act genuinely interested in their work.

8. **Set a good example**: As your child sees you focus on your work and practice all these suggested tips; they are more likely to follow your example and accept your guidance.

9. **If there are ongoing struggles, get help**: Talk with your student's teacher. Talk to friends, relatives, other parents, or the school counselor.

10. **Celebrate success**: Achievements are prime motivators and often remembered forever. Affirming a student's abilities builds their confidence. When your praise is sincere, specific and relevant to your student's achievement they can become very inspired. Simple gestures such as a greeting card, a complimentary phone call or a favorite treat can go a long way towards support for your student's long-term success.

About the Authors

Gary Ficek earned a bachelor degree in Business Management and a master's degree in Engineering Management, Omega Rho, from Portland State University. He holds several professional certifications, including the Project Management Institutes Agile Certified Practitioner (PMI-ACP), Project Management Professional (PMP), Lean Six Sigma Blackbelt (LSSBB), Prosci Change Management, and Kaizen Leader. He has also managed multi-million-dollar construction projects, process improvement, and strategic initiatives programs for over 20 years. Gary is a US Army veteran having served as team leader with the 75th Ranger Regiment and as a member of a US Special Forces A-team.

At the time of this writing, Alan Ficek was in the 7th grade. He was born in July and has always been one of the youngest students in his class; but this has never stopped Alan from always doing his best and never giving up. He played Little League baseball for six years as a catcher, pitcher and outfielder. He is now learning to drive shifter karts and the sweet science of boxing. Math and science are Alan's favorite school subjects. Like his father, Alan is an outdoorsman and has true grit.